Skin Care

EXPRESS

Skin Care Express

Skin Care

EXPRESS

Know How to Take Care of Your Skin

Rhonda Fields & KnowIt Express

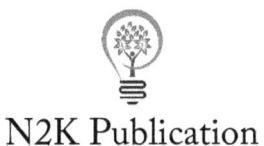

N2K Publication

ISBN 978-1-535-31732-0

Printed in the United States of America

First Edition

Welcome to the *Know It Express* - the express lane to knowledge!

To stay up-to-date, please be sure to sign up for **our newsletter** at http://www.KnowItExpress.com and follow us on social media:

https://www.facebook.com/KnowItExpress
https://twitter.com/KnowItExpress
https://plus.google.com/+KnowItExpress

Skin Care Express

EXPRESS LANE

Skin Care Express

CHAPTER 1

Searching for the Fountain of Youth

Beauty In The Skin

Everyone admires a god or goddess when they see one, right? You know what makes them stand out?

FLAWLESS SKIN!!!

Since the dawn of civilization, the obsession with staying young and beautiful has led some on a quest for the Fountain of Youth to the creation of other superstitious beliefs. This shows the great length people will go to achieve everlasting beauty.

But it's all understandable.

The need for healthy and beautiful skin cannot be overemphasized. Some of the reasons you should begin to take your skin seriously (other than for attracting the ladies or gents) are:

- Outer body defense mechanism
- Health and attraction indicators
- Acceptance and professional progression

Outer Body Defense Mechanism

Your skin is your body's primary defense mechanism.

For those who love knowledge, and specifically for those with an interest in biology, if you didn't already know, there are billions of micro-organisms in the atmosphere.

Without healthy skin, your body will no longer be able to host the benign and codependent organisms without being attacked by the malignant variety. The harmful organisms will penetrate under your skin and seek out your internal organs where they will wreak havoc on your entire system.

There's little wonder why it's advised to treat skin cuts right away to avoid infections.

When the skin is not properly cared for, the population of the harmful organisms will surpass the beneficial properties of the other organisms residing in your skin. This is when you run into trouble.

The skin is also the fastest vehicle to the spread of many communicable diseases.

Health And Attraction Indicators

Having beautiful skin is a sign of health.

Imagine what would happen if someone sat down next to you who smelled like they hadn't showered for a month, or better still, imagine someone with obvious rashes and sores approaching you with open arms.

You would be anywhere from uncomfortable to horrified and disgusted, right?

Skin abnormalities, such as eczema and acne, can result in social rejection. But even with wider acceptance of skin disorders, the appearance of your skin may be the very reason why your dream job still eludes you.

Although you can't change your genetics, you can improve the appearance of your skin to get people to want to stick around...because hey, being around attractive people makes others appear more attractive themselves by power of association.

Society does take notice if your skin is unpleasant to behold.

Acceptance And Professional Progression

Besides the health implications, your healthy and beautiful skin is also important when you're pursuing a career or just milling about in the general public.

- Take for example: Modeling. Your job is to look good and make love to the camera alright, but the end goal is to sell lots and lots of stuff, from clothes and accessories adorning your body to luxury items or everyday goods like health products and even foods. This way you are like an ambassador for your clients who are paying you big bucks to appeal to their targeted prospects. Believe it or not, there are people who would buy, not because of the products themselves, but because they admire your radiant skin. If, as a model, your skin turns off your viewers, how do you think they will approach your brand? With disgust, right?

OK, enough with the modeling example. Let's be honest, people have a natural inclination to choose better-looking people than those who are less polished in their appearance.

Remember the good old cliché "dress to impress"?

So make your skin healthy and beautiful for both yourself and others. This will enhance your already stylish presentation.

CHAPTER 2

Caring for Different Skin Types

Custom Skin Regimens

Now we come to address the question you've been waiting for: how can you get healthy and beautiful skin?

To start off, everyone's skin is unique – color, type, texture, and more. So what may be a problem for one person's skin may not be an issue for someone else.

There are various skin types: normal, dry, oily, sensitive.

Though a small tilt to each skin type may not be much of a problem, extremes of each may be both unbearable and uncomfortable to the individual.

What follows next explains each skin type and the proper care for them.

Normal Skin Care

Normal skin may not be much of a problem. The 'normal' here is simply referring to skin that has just the right amount of oil (and not necessarily the absence of black heads, wrinkles and some other common skin defects).

You can regard your skin as normal if:

- Formulations of oily skin cause you dryness and that of dry skin makes you greasy.

- Most parts of your body remain unchanged (neither dry nor greasy) for most of the day.

- You don't see the need to dab your skin and apply powder frequently or splash on a moisturizer during the day.

If you already have normal skin, then you must avoid heavy moisturizers. Stick with mild soaps. (Baby soaps work just as well.)

For normal skin suffering from wrinkles, there is a bit of concern because wrinkles need some level of hydration. Bearing in mind that hydration can cause greasiness in normal skin, what is the next step?

For normal skin struggling with wrinkles, try a moisture-based cleanser that will hydrate without causing oil in your skin. Oil-based moisturizers are not recommended.

- Get your moisture-based cleanser.

- Dip a cotton ball into the cleanser and use the cotton to massage the area gently in a circular motion (wrinkles mostly occur under the eyes, forehead and corners of the mouth).

- Allow the moisture to dry before applying your makeup.

Also, resist advanced skin replenishing toners and daily smoothing treatments with alpha hydroxy acids (AHA).

If oil-based hydrating creams or lotions must be used, then only use them at night.

Oily Skin Care

Oily skin can be problematic, especially if you're wearing makeup. It won't take long before the oil taints your makeup and makes it run. *Not very attractive, eh?* Yet on a positive note, the oil coming from your skin will keep you healthier by choking off the harmful organisms trying to seep past.

Fortunately, there are many ways to cut down on body oil. According to April Armstrong, MD, a dermatologist at the University of California, Davis, said that it is better to use gentle cleansers because harsh soaps trigger the skin to produce more oil.

Cleansers with acids such as benzoyl peroxide, salicylic acid, glycolic acid, or beta-hydroxy acid have been proven by dermatologists to be good for cutting down oils. If your basic cleanser is not working, you can go for a product with one of those. No matter what you do, always avoid products that cause clogging of the pores.

The steps you would need to control oily skin are:

- Use a water-soluble cleanser that doesn't have a drying agent such as sodium lauryl sulfate.

- Use an alcohol-free toner to get rid of dead skin cells, which often clogs the skin. Antioxidants in toners help to reduce inflammation.

- Exfoliate! It opens up your pores. Salicylic acid is the best for oily skin. Continued use will also help to fade away old blemishes.

- Hydrate with non-pore-clogging creams. But only do this before bed. It will help in your wrinkle-prevention plan.

Dry Skin Care

There are certain regions in the world where the water evaporates into the atmosphere leaving the surrounding area exceptionally dry. This can be a serious problem for those with dry skin. Not only does the texture become flaky, it becomes brittle as well. Brittle skin breaks with little stimulation. This can cause irritation and pain as well as a lower social status depending on where and how bad the cuts are.

A lack of hydration causes wrinkles, so hydration is key to healthy skin for this specific skin type.

But don't worry, there are a few things you can do to salvage the situation and bring your skin type closer to normal.

Hot water feels good on the skin when the weather is chilly, right? But what you may not know is that water higher than 40 degrees will dissolve the oil barriers in your skin. All that oil protecting your skin will circle down the drain with your bath water. You know what that means? More dryness.

You can deal with this issue using the following techniques:

- Take a bath with warm water instead of hot (bath should not exceed 15 minutes).

- After bathing, resist the temptation to rub yourself with a towel, rather, dab your skin with it.

- If you must shave, do it in the shower or immediately afterwards. The hairs are softer then and there will be less irritation to the skin.

- Use lots of moisturizers. Moisturizers will help your skin retain moisture and keep wrinkling in check.

Sensitive Skin Care

Sensitive skin is another type of skin that can go hand-in-hand with any of the three prior skin types. You can call it "the mother of them all." The symptoms of sensitive skin include such things as rashes, redness, itching, puffiness and so on.

Sensitive skin is often an indication of sudden changes; your skin telling you that you are not doing something right. Though some people are born with natural allergies, when you start witnessing some of the symptoms mentioned above, it may be an environmental factor or be related to something else external: chemical or gas in the air or from your cosmetics.

When your skin blushes on sudden impact or as a result of temperature changes, it may be an indication that you are suffering from rosacea. Topically applying metronidazole or taking oral tetracycline is known to be very effective. The cause is not known, but is more common among middle-aged and elderly women.

Prolonged use of anti-aging creams and skin bleaching agents will normally upset the skin melanin and other strengthening agents, making it more sensitive.

If your skin is irritated, do the following:

- Scrub lightly during your shower to avoid irritated skin.

- Limit your intake of alcohol.

- Try to detect the ingredient in your creams that causes the irritation and avoid them.

- Don't go to grassy areas and also avoid items that can cause itching.

<u>Exercise</u>: What's Your Skin Type

You have gone through the various skin types. Now it's time for you to identify yours.

1.) Observe your skin (face and arms) for 24 hours without applying anything.

2.) Write down what you noticed (oily, dry, no change).

3.) Repeat for another 24 hours with heavy creams and report.

4.) By now you should have an idea of your skin type. (You may even notice you have a combination of symptoms from more than one skin-type.)

CHAPTER 3

Rejuvenating Your Skin

It Goes Beyond The Surface

Look in the mirror? Yikes? Don't panic. The world isn't coming to an end just because you may be dealing with wrinkles, blackheads, and acne. You can still awaken your skin and give it that youthful look you always desired or missed.

The truth about your skin is that what goes on inside of you, will most often be reflected on the outside of you...through your skin.

Therefore, to rejuvenate your skin, you will need to begin from the inside-out.

Nutrition Builds Up Your Skin

When it comes to skin care, what goes into the mouth matters!

Chain-smoking and drinking alcohol cause the body to stop carrying out its natural repairs. Not only that, but alcohol causes your body to burn fat at a faster rate, which causes wrinkles.

Instead of alcohol, go for plenty of water. Water keeps the skin hydrated and supple.

Fruits are very beneficial because of their high content of antioxidants and some even have a lot of vitamin C as well. In fact, you can get vitamin C from both fruits and vegetables. The ones with the highest concentrations are bell peppers, berries, broccoli, citrus fruits, dark leafy greens, kiwis, papayas, peas, and tomatoes. Anything with a high concentration of vitamin C can stave off or even reverse the pesky issue of scurvy.

If you have swollen gums, a rash of tiny bleeding spots, and cracked and bleeding skin around the mouth, then make sure to eat plenty of the yummy foods mentioned above.

For skin rejuvenation, also go for lots of leafy vegetables because of their iron deposits. As you may already know, iron is needed for blood formation. The fresher the blood in your body, the higher your chances of a healthier skin.

Get The Blood Flowing Through Your Skin

Exercise should be part of your daily life, not pushed off to the side. Your skin needs it! Have you ever seen athletes' skin? They rarely seem to age. The secret? Exercise!!!

There are two types of exercise you can choose – aerobic and anaerobic. The biggest difference is the intensity at which you perform these exercises.

- Aerobic exercise should increase your heart rate and your breathing, but not so much that you can't sustain the activity. Aerobic literally translates to 'with oxygen.' An example of aerobic exercise is biking around your neighborhood.

- Anaerobic, on the other hand, means 'without oxygen.' This is when you get out of breath in just a few minutes. An example of anaerobic exercise is biking in the Tour de France alongside Lance Armstrong.

Always keep in mind that the less you worry, the slower you age.

Why They Called It 'Beauty Sleep'

Whether you're working hard or having massive amounts of fun, don't over do it to the point that it deprives you of the proper amount of sleep.

Here's an example:

If you have a cut on your thumb but continue with a heavy workload, does the wound clot easily? Of course not. You know what does help? You guessed it – sleep! During rest and sleep, the flow of blood becomes gentle and the muscles also relax making it easier for worn tissues to heal themselves.

If you are suffering from insomnia, there are some techniques to help you sleep besides medication – this is not always the best option when you consider the side effects.

- A cup of milk or yogurt helps to calm the nerves, so consider taking one before going to bed.

- Switch off all the lights. The presence of light makes the nerves uneasy. Once you begin to have proper rest, you will notice your skin texture begin to improve.

Mind Your Hygiene

When it comes to overall well-being, personal hygiene is everything.

In terms of skin care, you should focus on:

How often and how thoroughly you bathe as well as how clean your clothes are.

Even if you do take care of your skin, your clothes could be the problem. They need to be:

- Properly washed after each use, particularly if you've been sweating

- Given enough time to dry

- Ironed

Exercise: Your Skin Maintenance

Having gone through the ways of improving your skin, the next big step would be to focus on behavioral changes. The best way to take good advice is to make it a part of you.

Some of the things you will need to do are:

- Prepare a personal timetable: a timetable will help you organize your life. In your timetable include: work hours, leisure time, meal times, and sleep. It should have three columns: days of the week, hours of the day, and activities. Most importantly: respect your timetable!

- You must have noticed the importance of water in keeping your skin hydrated and supple. Make it part of your daily routine to carry a plastic bottle of water wherever you go. It's to remind you to always keep yourself hydrated.

CHAPTER 4

Protecting Your Skin from the Environment

You Scratch My Back, I Scratch Yours

Your relationship with your skin should be mutual.

As much as the skin protects you, there are times you will need to protect your skin too. An example is when you're in an environment of extreme heat or extreme cold.

In extreme cold, fat deposits beneath the skin work to cover up your pores in order to keep you warm. If the skin is not aided with thick clothing, the cells close to the skin will begin to freeze and burst open. This is what they call frostbite. Extreme cases of frostbite can lead to amputation of the affected area.

Best Line Of Defense Against Aging

When it comes to taking care of your skin, the importance of sun safety cannot be emphasized enough. You probably already know the harshness of sunlight on the skin can cause sunburns and skin cancer, right?

The sun produces UVA, UVB and UVC rays. UVA and UVB rays bring that beautiful summer glow, but it also causes premature aging of the skin. Who doesn't love a tan, but is it really worth it?

Put on a hat when walking in the sun since it provides a barrier against those damaging rays. And when you're at the beach, make sure to apply sunscreen often. No one wants to get burned. Ouch!

In order to prevent wrinkles, it's vital to wear a broad-spectrum sunscreen everyday with an SPF of 30 or more. Make sure the sunscreen you choose is geared towards your skin type. Fifteen minutes before going out in the sun, make sure to apply your sunscreen. This is the single best defense against premature aging of your skin and it prevents skin cancer. Nice!

It is also important to mention vitamin C usage here. Topical application of vitamin C before sun exposure has been linked to increased protection from the sun. Vitamin C also helps to treat pigmentation, brightens the complexion, and helps in the production of collagen, the building block of our skin and the compound that gives our skin it's suppleness.

CHAPTER 5

Enhancing Your Skin

Get Evenly-Toned Skin

An uneven skin tone can also make you a social pariah.

- One reason this happens is when your clothes are too tight. One of the most prominent examples is when women wear bikinis. The areas exposed to the sun are much darker, while the part of the skin covered by the swimsuit is much lighter.

The best way to even out your skin tone is by ingesting antioxidants, such as blueberries and pomegranates. Exercise also improves blood flow. Better blood flow results in a more even skin tone. These solutions are more long lasting than trying to fix the problem with lotions.

Massage your skin daily. But if you're too busy, then once a week is fine. Massage helps blood to flow better in the capillaries and also relaxes the muscles.

After one week of massage, use exfoliating creams to get rid of dead skin. Dead skin cells have a tendency to trap skin oils. These trapped skin oils will then mix with other waste components, which forms a hard mass that oxidizes in the presence of oxygen to cause blackheads. You can make your own exfoliating cream.

1.) Get one cup of honey.

2.) Add two to three tablespoons of sugar, syrup or honey with white oats.

3.) Mix and rub on the area you want to exfoliate.

4.) Keep on for twenty to thirty minutes and wash off.

The Magic Of Makeup

Makeup is a brilliant way to have an even skin tone and also hide blemishes.

Makeup gives you similar powers like the popular editing software, Photoshop. With makeup, you can tweak your looks to almost how you want it. You know why movie stars look different on the big screen compared to their looks in everyday life?

Why, makeup, of course.

The hard work you did to find out your skin type will come in handy when you opt for makeup to augment your look. Your makeup procedure will differ substantially based on your skin type. For example, if you have oily skin, your makeup kit should contain drying agents (ex. matte), while dry skin should have a kit with lots of moisturizers.

The following steps should help you find the perfect makeup to compliment your skin tone:

- **Shower.** The first step to makeup is to have a proper bath. A shower washes away dirt and excess oils on the surface of the skin. The dirt and oils will decrease the amount of time the makeup will remain on your skin.

- **Foundation.** This is where people get it wrong. Some think foundation doesn't really matter, but it really does! Without a good foundation, skin oils will slip out of the skin and taint your makeup. Apply one light layer of foundation to your skin and make sure you can blend it seamlessly based on your skin tone. This will help even your skin tone so that the rest of the makeup you apply looks flawless.

- **Concealer.** This is what erases those blemishes and ugly marks on your face. It conceals them and makes them fade away.

- **Blush.** This makes your cheekbones more prominent and gives your face better definition than if you didn't have it on.

- **Lipstick and Mascara.** These do not really aid your skin, but they can be used to enhance your face. When you use sharp colors on your lips and eyelashes, it will draw people's attention away from your body to your face.

The good thing about makeup is that once you are using the right one for your skin type, there are usually no side effects because they are superficial.

On the other hand, keep in mind that makeup is a cover-up, not a long-term solution. Makeup can get pricey if you're a fanatic, so pace yourself.

Excessive makeup will wear the skin down over time, so keep the makeup to a minimum. Be aware of the chemical and expiration dates on them; doing otherwise can do more harm than good.

CHAPTER 6

Maintaining Your Skin for Years to Come

The Effect Of Aging

By now you should have already determined your skin type: normal, oily, dry, sensitive, or a combination of these.

Here's a general guide to assist you on the aging process of what your skin goes through throughout the years of your life:

During Your 20's

If you are in your 20's, your focus should be on a good skin care routine that helps your skin stay moisturized.

You should be diligent with sunscreen use if you want to avoid the wrinkly, leathery look later on in your life.

Use a good eye cream that also has some anti-aging properties. Anti-aging and vitamin C serums will help you combat the early signs of aging. Add these to your normal routine.

During Your 30's

During your 30's, you tend to become more concerned with avoiding the signs of aging on your skin.

Fatigue and stress can start to show up on your face so try to keep yourself relaxed.

Start a good anti-aging regimen with a good moisturizer that also has anti-aging properties. Like always, use sunscreen like your life depends on it!

Get yourself a good eye cream that combats signs of aging and pamper yourself with spa days whenever you feel stressed.

Finally, keep using that vitamin C serum for a brighter complexion.

During Your 40's

During your 40's, you most likely have seen a few signs of aging.

It's best to start using products geared towards the treatment of wrinkles and age spots. You have many options in the market these days.

Use richer eye creams that help you fight wrinkles that you may be noticing these days.

Also keep up with regular exfoliation – particularly products that contain glycolic acids and vitamin C – because they help to regenerate lost collagen in your skin. With this regimen, you can get back the fullness you once had.

50+ And Mature Skin

During this time, many people focus on getting treatments for wrinkles and age spots – starting a topical prescription-strength retinoid to treat these.

Also, get regular glycolic acid peels, which also helps to regenerate the lost youthful look of your skin.

Your skin may be drier now than it was before, so always use moisturizers.

Final Last Resort

If you really are unhappy with the way your skin looks, then you always have the option of getting surgical help from a professional. These procedures provide you with endless skin rejuvenation possibilities.

Say you have been very careless in your youth and now cannot go back to fix the damage, what can you do to change your appearance for the better?

There are many options available these days including eyelid surgeries, brow lifts, face-lifts, neck lifts, fillers etc.

- If you are unhappy with the appearance of your eyes, for example, you can seek professional help to get an eyelid surgery done that will get rid of excess skin, giving you a more youthful look.

- Botox, made popular by celebrities, helps hide the appearance of wrinkles.

- A face-lift will literally lift your face to make you look younger and will get rid of any deep lines you may have.

A plastic surgeon will be your best guide when it comes to what works best for your face.

CHAPTER 7

Letting Your Skin Shine

Not So Skin Deep After All

The skin plays a dual role as the largest organ in the human body – it covers the other vital organs, and it is an excretory organ on its own.

Hence, your diet greatly affects the health of your skin. When your diet produces the kind of waste that labors the skin to excrete, the skin begins to age with its most visible sign being wrinkling.

Also, your skin needs to be protected from extreme temperatures, which kills your skin cells and causes you to look older than you are.

There are different skin types and the first step to skin care and treatment is to discover which category your skin falls into. Without this knowledge, you may be applying the wrong solution and instead of getting the desired result, you will be more frustrated.

Love Your Own Skin

No skin type is actually better than the other because everybody has different skin, but it is the way you manage what you have that matters. Therefore, instead of grieving for what you don't have, find and polish the gold in what you do.

Remember, life is too short to be spent staring in the mirror all day and wishing you had flawless skin.

Instead, do something about it! Start taking care for your skin today!

Skin Care Express

Now You Know!

We have now gone from - *NOT knowing*...to *KNOWING*.

Doesn't it feel great? As cliché as the proverbial saying goes: knowledge is, indeed, power. The more you know, the more empowered you become. Not knowing is defeating, as you succumb to feelings of helplessness and surrendering of your own self.

Of course, acquiring knowledge is a never-ending quest. There is a great saying by Nobel Prize French author Andre Gide: "Believe those who are seeking the truth. Doubt those who find it."

At the very least, we hope we have set you off in the right path in regards to what you have set out to know, and that you have enjoyed our little journey together for the time you have spent with us.

If you can tell us how we did, that would be very appreciated! We value your feedback and always look forward to hearing from you, or if there is any way we could improve the entire experience for you. If you have a success story, even better - please let us know!

http://www.KnowItExpress.com

Don't forget to stay in contact for we would love to connect with you.

https://www.facebook.com/KnowItExpress
https://twitter.com/KnowItExpress
https://plus.google.com/+KnowItExpress

What would you like to know? Let us know!

CONTACT US

Now onward for more power to you, and thank you!

Skin Care Express